FREEDOM REGAINED: THE BEST METHODS FOR QUITTING SMOKING

Sylvain MILON

SUMMARY

INTRODUCTION

Freedom Regained: The Best Methods for Quitting Smoking is a comprehensive and practical guide to help smokers break free from their addiction to tobacco. This book covers all aspects of the quitting process, providing practical advice, effective strategies and evidence-based information.

The introductory chapter outlines the dangers of smoking and the adverse health consequences, providing an awareness of the risks involved. The book then encourages readers to make the decision to quit smoking by highlighting the many benefits of quitting. It also explains why it is essential to set realistic goals and prepare mentally before beginning the quitting process.

In the following chapters, different methods of quitting smoking are explored in detail. Readers are guided through options such as nicotine replacement therapy, cognitive behavioral therapy, acupuncture, and other alternative approaches. Each method is presented objectively, providing information about its effectiveness and the scientific evidence that supports it.

The book also discusses withdrawal symptoms and offers practical advice on how to manage them effectively. It emphasizes the importance of building motivation and willpower, as well as preventing relapse by avoiding common pitfalls. Social and family support is also discussed, highlighting the importance of a supportive environment during the quitting process.

Finally, the book offers tips for adopting new healthy habits and managing stress and emotions without resorting to tobacco. It concludes by providing strategies for maintaining freedom and preventing long-term relapse.

This practical guide, backed by scientific research, is designed to give smokers the tools and knowledge they need to successfully quit smoking. Whether you are an occasional smoker or a long-time smoker, "Freedom Regained: The Best Methods for Quitting Smoking" is your ally for a life without tobacco.

CHAPTER 1: THE DANGERS OF SMOKING

Smoking is a common habit throughout the world, but it is essential to understand the many dangers that smokers face. In this chapter, we will explore the negative health effects of smoking, highlighting the risks to smokers and those around them.

1.1 Tobacco related diseases

Smoking is closely associated with many serious diseases that can have a significant impact on the quality of life of smokers. One of the most well-known consequences is cancer. Smoking is the leading cause of lung cancer, but it is also linked to other types of cancer such as those of the mouth, throat, esophagus, bladder and pancreas. Toxic substances in cigarette smoke damage cells and promote tumor formation.

In addition to cancer, smoking is a major risk factor for cardiovascular disease. The chemicals in cigarette smoke contribute to the buildup of fatty plaques in the arteries, which can lead to problems such as atherosclerosis, heart attacks, strokes and high blood pressure.

1.2 Effects on the respiratory system

Smoking has a significant impact on the respiratory system. Smokers are more likely to develop conditions such as chronic bronchitis and emphysema, grouped under the term chronic obstructive pulmonary disease (COPD). These diseases make it difficult to breathe, cause persistent coughing and lead to decreased lung capacity. Smokers also have an increased risk of respiratory infections such as pneumonia and acute bronchitis.

1.3 Impact on the health of others

Smoking not only affects the health of smokers, but also those around them. Exposure to second-hand smoke, also known as passive smoking, poses serious health risks. Non-smokers who inhale second-hand smoke are exposed to the same toxic substances as smokers. This can lead to respiratory problems, cardiovascular disease and increased susceptibility to infections.

In addition, pregnant women who smoke or are exposed to second-hand smoke are at risk to their own health and that of their babies. Smoking during pregnancy is associated with an increased risk of complications such as premature birth, miscarriage, low birth weight and birth defects.

1.4 Nicotine addiction

Tobacco contains nicotine, a highly addictive substance. When inhaled, nicotine quickly reaches the brain and creates a physical and psychological dependency. Smokers feel the need to smoke to satisfy their nicotine cravings, making it extremely difficult to quit.

Nicotine dependence is one of the biggest obstacles to quitting smoking. Withdrawal symptoms such as irritability, anxiety, sleep disturbances and intense cravings can make the quitting process particularly difficult. However, it is important to understand that nicotine addiction can be overcome with the right methods and support.

In conclusion, smoking presents many health hazards. Smokers are at increased risk of developing serious diseases such as cancer, cardiovascular disease and lung disease. In addition, smoking also affects the health of non-smokers, especially those who are exposed to second-hand smoke. It is therefore important to be aware of these dangers and to take steps to break free from tobacco addiction. In the following chapters, we will explore the best ways to quit smoking and return to a smoke-free life of health and freedom.

CHAPTER 2: MAKING THE DECISION TO QUIT

Making the decision to quit smoking is an essential step toward a healthier, more fulfilling life. In this chapter, we will explore the different motivations that can lead to this decision, the benefits of quitting smoking and the potential obstacles you may encounter.

2.1 Finding your motivation

The first step in quitting smoking is to find your own motivation. Everyone has different reasons for quitting, whether it's concern for your health, preserving your relationships, improving your appearance or protecting your loved ones from second-hand smoke. Take some time to think about what really motivates you to quit smoking.

It may be helpful to make a list of the benefits of quitting smoking. Think about your health and improved quality of life. Also consider the financial savings you could realize by quitting smoking. The more motivated you are, the easier it will be to face the challenges ahead.

2.2 The benefits of quitting smoking

Quitting smoking has many benefits for your health and well-being. First of all, your health will improve considerably. Your lungs will get rid of the toxic substances present in cigarette smoke, which will allow you to breathe better and reduce respiratory problems. Your risk of developing serious diseases such as cancer, cardiovascular disease and lung disease will gradually decrease.

By quitting smoking, you will also regain a healthier skin and a more radiant complexion. Cigarette smoke contributes to premature skin aging, wrinkles and a dull complexion. By quitting smoking, you will promote better blood circulation, which will result in improved skin appearance.

Quitting smoking will also have a positive impact on your social relationships. You will no longer be bothered by the smell of smoke on your clothes and breath, which will boost your confidence and self-esteem. In addition, you will protect your loved ones from the dangers of second-hand smoke, which will help to preserve their health.

2.3 Barriers to Smoking Cessation

While there are many benefits to quitting smoking, it is important to recognize the potential barriers you may face. Nicotine dependence is one of the biggest obstacles to quitting smoking. Withdrawal symptoms such as irritability, anxiety, sleep disturbances and intense cravings can make the quitting process difficult.

You may also encounter stressful situations or moments that make you want to light up a cigarette. Identify these moments and prepare yourself to deal with them by implementing stress management strategies and healthy alternatives to distract yourself.

The influence of your social environment can also be a challenge. If you are surrounded by smokers or frequent places where smoking is common, it may be harder to resist the temptation. Communicate with those around you and ask them to support you in your efforts to quit smoking.

In conclusion, making the decision to quit smoking is a courageous act that will benefit your health. Find your own motivation and focus on the benefits of quitting. Be aware of potential obstacles and be prepared to overcome them. In the following chapters, we will explore the most effective methods and strategies to help you achieve your goal of a tobacco-free life.

CHAPTER 3: SETTING REALISTIC GOALS

When you decide to quit smoking, it is important to set realistic and achievable goals. In this chapter, we will explore the importance of setting clear goals, the benefits of making them realistic, and strategies for achieving them.

3.1 The importance of setting clear objectives

Setting clear goals is essential to your success in quitting smoking. A clear goal gives you a clear direction and allows you to measure your progress. Instead of just saying "I want to quit smoking," set specific, measurable goals such as "I will quit smoking in the next three weeks" or "I will cut my cigarette consumption in half by the end of the month.

Having clear goals will keep you motivated and focused on your quitting journey. You can even break down your main goal into smaller, more achievable sub-goals. This will give you a series of small victories that will boost your confidence and encourage you to keep trying.

3.2 The benefits of setting realistic goals

Setting realistic goals is crucial to maintaining your motivation and avoiding feelings of frustration and failure. It is important to recognize that quitting smoking is an individual process and that it can vary from person to person. Setting goals that are too ambitious or unrealistic can create undue pressure and demoralize you if you don't achieve them.

By setting realistic goals, you give yourself a real chance to achieve them and celebrate your progress. For example, if you are a regular smoker, setting a goal of gradually reducing your cigarette consumption instead of quitting cold turkey may be more realistic and effective for you.

3.3 Strategies to achieve your goals

To achieve your quit smoking goals, it is important to have effective strategies in place. Here are some tips to help you:

1. Plan your quit: Set a specific date to quit smoking. Prepare yourself mentally and physically by identifying situations or habits related to smoking that you will need to change.

2. Seek support: Tell those around you about your decision to quit smoking and ask for their support. You may also want to consider joining support groups or seeing a health care professional who specializes in smoking cessation.

3. Use nicotine replacement products: Nicotine replacement products such as patches, gum or inhalers can help relieve withdrawal symptoms and gradually reduce your nicotine dependence.

4. Adopt new habits: Identify the times or activities that cause you to smoke and replace them with new healthy habits. For example, if you used to smoke after meals, try taking a short walk instead.

5. Deal with cravings: Cravings can be intense, but they are temporary. Use relaxation techniques, such as deep breathing, to help you overcome them. Distracting your mind by doing something you are passionate about can also be effective.

By setting realistic goals and implementing the right strategies, you will increase your chances of quitting successfully. Remember, every step toward a smoke-free life is a victory in itself. In the following chapters, we'll explore more techniques and tips to help you reach your goals and break free from tobacco addiction for good.

CHAPTER 4:
PREPARING MENTALLY

Mental preparation is an essential part of successfully quitting smoking. In this chapter, we will explore the importance of mental preparation, strategies for building motivation and resilience, and techniques for dealing with negative thoughts.

4.1 The importance of mental preparation

Mental preparation is essential to deal with the challenges and temptations that can arise when quitting smoking. Nicotine addiction is both physical and psychological, so it is crucial to be prepared to deal with withdrawal symptoms and cravings.

Mental preparation involves developing a positive attitude, self-confidence and strong motivation to succeed in quitting smoking. It involves understanding why you want to quit, visualizing your life without tobacco and taking a proactive approach to the difficulties that may arise.

4.2 Building motivation and resilience

Strengthening your motivation and stamina is essential to staying committed to your quit journey. Here are some strategies for doing so:

- Identify your motivations: Spend some time thinking about why you want to quit smoking. What are the benefits to your health, appearance, relationships or finances? Write them down and review them when you need a motivating reminder.

- Visualize your success: Imagine yourself living a tobacco-free life, in full health and in control of your choices. Visualize yourself facing and successfully overcoming situations where you would normally smoke. This positive visualization boosts your motivation and confidence.

- Surround yourself with support: Seek out support from family, friends or support groups that specialize in quitting smoking. Sharing your goals with others who understand what you are going through can help you stay motivated and get through the tough times.

4.3 Dealing with negative thoughts

During the quitting process, it is common to experience negative thoughts or doubts about your ability to succeed. It is important to develop strategies to deal with these thoughts and turn them into positive, constructive thoughts.

- Identify negative thoughts: Be aware of negative thoughts that arise when you are faced with a craving or difficulty in quitting. Identify these thoughts and replace them with positive ones. For example, instead of saying to yourself, "I can't do it," say to yourself, "I can overcome this urge and lead a smoke-free life.

- Use positive affirmations: Create positive affirmations and repeat them regularly to build your confidence. For example, say to yourself, "I am strong and I can quit smoking" or "I am taking care of my health by choosing to live tobacco-free".

- Practice mindfulness: Mindfulness is a technique that involves being fully aware of the present moment without judgment. When you feel a craving or a negative thought, take a few moments to focus on your breathing, observe your thoughts without attachment and let them pass. Mindfulness helps you step back from your thoughts and develop a more positive and detached attitude.

By preparing yourself mentally, building motivation and resilience, and dealing with negative thoughts, you will be better prepared to successfully quit smoking. Mental preparation is an important key to overcoming the challenges that can arise during the quitting process. In the following chapters, we will explore more strategies and tools to help you achieve your goals and live a tobacco-free life.

CHAPTER 5:
CHOOSING THE RIGHT
METHOD FOR YOU

When you decide to quit smoking, there are many methods available to help you along the way. In this chapter, we'll explore the different smoking cessation options, the pros and cons of each method, and tips for choosing the one that's right for you.

5.1 Smoking Cessation Options

There are several smoking cessation options to choose from. Here are the most common methods:

- Quitting cold turkey: This involves quitting smoking overnight, without using nicotine replacement products. This method requires a strong will and a solid mental preparation, but it can be very effective for some people.

- Nicotine replacement products: Nicotine replacement products, such as patches, gum, inhalers or chewable tablets, provide a controlled dose of nicotine to relieve withdrawal symptoms. They can help you gradually reduce your dependence on nicotine.

- Prescription medications: There are prescription medications, such as varenicline (Champix) or bupropion (Zyban), that can help reduce cravings and withdrawal symptoms. These medications work on the nicotine receptors in your brain.

- Behavioral therapy: Behavioral therapy is an approach to changing your smoking-related behaviors and habits. It may include techniques such as stress management, cognitive restructuring and positive reinforcement.

5.2 Advantages and disadvantages of the different methods

Each smoking cessation method has advantages and disadvantages that are important to consider when choosing the method that is best for you.

- Cold turkey: The advantage of this method is that it allows you to stop quickly and decisively. However, withdrawal symptoms can be more intense, and it takes a great deal of willpower to maintain this stop without external support.

- Nicotine Substitutes: Nicotine substitutes offer a milder alternative by providing a controlled dose of nicotine to relieve withdrawal symptoms. However, they can prolong nicotine dependence and require regular and appropriate use.

- Prescription drugs: Prescription drugs can be effective in reducing cravings, but they can have side effects and should be used under medical supervision.

- Behavioral therapy: Behavioral therapy addresses the

psychological and behavioral aspects of tobacco addiction. It can be effective in the long term, but it requires commitment and active participation.

5.3 Tips for choosing the right method for you

To help you choose the best smoking cessation method for you, here are some tips:

- Consult a health care professional: Talk to a doctor, pharmacist or smoking cessation specialist for advice tailored to your situation and needs.

- Consider your personal preferences: Think about your preferences in terms of method of cessation, mode of administration (patches, gum, etc.) and desired support.

- Assess your habits and addiction: Consider your level of nicotine addiction, smoking habits and triggers. Some methods may be better suited to your specific needs.

- Be prepared to adjust your approach: You may need to try different methods or combine several approaches to find what works best for you.

By choosing the smoking cessation method that works best for you, you increase your chances of success in quitting smoking. Remember, there is no one-size-fits-all method that works for everyone, and it's important to find the one that works for you personally. In the following chapters, we will discuss more strategies and tips to help you on your journey to a tobacco-free life.

CHAPTER 6: NICOTINE SUBSTITUTES

Nicotine replacement products are products designed to help smokers quit by providing a controlled dose of nicotine. In this chapter, we will explore the different types of nicotine replacement products available, how they work, and the advantages and disadvantages of using them.

6.1 The different types of nicotine replacement products

There are several types of nicotine replacement products that you can choose from depending on your preferences and needs. Here are the main types:

- Patches: Patches are adhesive devices that you apply to your skin. They slowly release nicotine into your body throughout the day. Patches are convenient because they do not require any special gesture and can be used discreetly.

- Chewing gums: Chewing gums are specially formulated chewing gums containing nicotine. You chew the gum and the nicotine is absorbed through the mucous membranes of the mouth. Chewing gum is convenient because it allows you to control your nicotine dose according to your needs.

- Inhalers: Inhalers are devices that look like electronic cigarettes. They contain a nicotine cartridge that you inhale, simulating the act of smoking. Inhalers offer a gestural alternative for smokers who need something to hold between their fingers.

- Sucking tablets: Sucking tablets are placed in the mouth and nicotine is released when they dissolve. They offer a discreet option and can be used in situations where chewing gum is not practical.

6.2 How nicotine replacement products work

Nicotine replacement products work by providing your body with a controlled amount of nicotine, without the other toxic substances found in cigarette smoke. They help relieve withdrawal symptoms and reduce cravings.

The nicotine in substitutes is absorbed into your body through the mucous membranes of your mouth, skin or lungs, depending on the type of substitute used. It then reaches your brain and binds to nicotine receptors, causing the release of dopamine, a neurotransmitter linked to pleasure and reward.

By providing a controlled dose of nicotine, nicotine replacement products help reduce withdrawal symptoms such as cravings, irritability and frustration. They also help break the link between nicotine and the habitual actions associated with smoking.

6.3 Advantages and disadvantages of nicotine replacement products

There are both advantages and disadvantages to using nicotine replacement therapy. Here is an overview of the main points to consider:

- Benefits:

  - Reduced withdrawal symptoms: Nicotine replacement products help reduce withdrawal symptoms such as cravings and irritability, making it easier to quit smoking.

  - Nicotine dose control: You can choose the dosage that matches your level of addiction and gradually reduce it over time.

  - Availability and accessibility: Nicotine replacement products are widely available over the counter in pharmacies and stores, making them easily accessible.

- Disadvantages:

  - Maintenance of nicotine dependence: The use of nicotine replacement products can prolong nicotine dependence, although in less harmful forms than cigarettes.

  - Possible side effects: Some users may experience side effects such as headache, nausea, mouth or skin irritation. These effects are usually temporary and disappear with time.

It is important to note that nicotine replacement products are not a quick fix, but they can be a valuable tool in your quitting journey. They can help you cope with withdrawal symptoms and gradually reduce your dependence on nicotine.

Before using nicotine replacement therapy, it is recommended that you consult a health care professional for advice tailored to your situation. In the following chapters, we will explore other strategies and tips to help you quit smoking and live a tobacco-free life.

CHAPTER 7: COGNITIVE BEHAVIORAL THERAPY

Cognitive behavioral therapy (CBT) is a psychological approach that has been shown to be effective in the smoking cessation process. In this chapter, we will explore the basic principles of CBT, its application in smoking cessation, and the techniques and tools used to help you overcome tobacco addiction.

7.1 Principles of Cognitive Behavioral Therapy

CBT is based on the idea that our thoughts, emotions and behaviors are interconnected. It aims to identify and change negative or irrational thought patterns that may contribute to tobacco addiction.

Here are some basic principles of CBT:

- Cognitive restructuring: This involves identifying negative automatic thoughts related to smoking and replacing them with positive, realistic thoughts. For example, instead of thinking, "I can never quit smoking," you can think, "I have the ability to quit smoking and I can succeed.

- Stress management: CBT teaches stress management techniques to help you cope with stressful situations without resorting to smoking. This may include relaxation exercises, deep breathing techniques or distraction activities.

- Positive Reinforcement: CBT focuses on reinforcing positive behaviors related to quitting smoking. This may include rewards for milestones or the use of self-reinforcement techniques, such as keeping a progress journal.

7.2 The application of CBT in smoking cessation

CBT can be used in many different ways to help you quit smoking. Here are some examples of how CBT can be used in smoking cessation:

- Identifying triggers: CBT helps you identify situations, emotions or habits that trigger the urge to smoke. By recognizing these triggers, you can develop strategies to avoid them or deal with them in a healthier way.

- Planning coping strategies: CBT helps you develop coping strategies to deal with cravings. This may include distraction techniques, use of nicotine replacement therapy, or adopting healthier alternative behaviors.

- Strengthening Resistance Skills: CBT teaches you to resist cravings by developing self-efficacy and resistance skills. This may include learning refusal techniques, repeating positive affirmations and identifying the benefits of quitting.

7.3 CBT Techniques and Tools for Smoking Cessation

CBT uses a variety of techniques and tools to help you quit smoking. Here are some common examples:

- Thought Journal: Keeping a thought journal allows you to record your thoughts about smoking and identify negative or irrational thought patterns. It helps you become aware of your thoughts and change them in a more positive way.

- Gradual Exposure: Gradual exposure is the controlled exposure to situations that trigger cravings to build tolerance and strengthen your resistance skills.

- Problem-solving training: This technique helps you identify problems related to quitting smoking and find effective solutions. It encourages exploring different options and developing an action plan to deal with obstacles.

CBT can be used alone or in combination with other smoking cessation methods, such as nicotine replacement therapy. It offers a comprehensive approach by targeting both the cognitive and behavioral aspects of tobacco addiction.

In conclusion, cognitive behavioral therapy is a powerful approach to helping you quit smoking. By working on your thoughts, feelings, and behaviors related to smoking, you can develop skills and strategies to overcome tobacco addiction. In the following chapters, we will explore other methods and tips to support you on your journey to quit smoking.

CHAPTER 8: ACUPUNCTURE AND OTHER ALTERNATIVE APPROACHES

In our quest to quit smoking, we are often willing to explore different approaches and methods. Acupuncture and other alternative approaches are among the options that some smokers consider to help them in their quest to quit. In this chapter, we will examine the effectiveness of acupuncture, as well as other alternative approaches, and discuss their use in the smoking cessation process.

8.1 Acupuncture: an ancient practice for quitting smoking

Acupuncture is a form of traditional Chinese medicine that involves the insertion of fine needles into specific points on the body. According to acupuncture theory, these acupuncture points are connected to energy meridians that can be stimulated to restore balance to the body. In the context of smoking cessation, acupuncture is often used to reduce withdrawal symptoms and cravings.

Some studies have suggested that acupuncture may be beneficial for people trying to quit smoking. For example, a study published in the Journal of the American Medical Association found that auricular acupuncture (ear acupuncture) was associated with a significant reduction in cravings in smokers who were trying to quit. However, other studies have produced mixed results and more research is needed to confirm the effectiveness of acupuncture in smoking cessation.

8.2 Alternative approaches to smoking cessation

In addition to acupuncture, there are other alternative approaches that are sometimes used in smoking cessation. Here are some of them:

- Hypnotherapy: Hypnotherapy uses hypnosis to help smokers change their behavior and thoughts about smoking. It can be used to increase motivation to quit smoking, reduce cravings and promote healthy lifestyle habits.

- Herbal therapy: Some herbs are known for their calming and relaxing properties, which can be beneficial for reducing stress and cravings. For example, passionflower, valerian and lemon balm are often used to help ease withdrawal symptoms.

- Group therapy and social support: Participating in support groups or group smoking cessation programs can provide emotional support, practical advice and the opportunity to share experiences with others in the same situation.

It is important to note that these alternative approaches may not be suitable for everyone, and their effectiveness may vary from person to person. It is recommended that you consult a health care professional or qualified practitioner to discuss alternative options and determine which ones may be most appropriate for you.

In conclusion, acupuncture and other alternative approaches can be considered as potential adjuncts in the smoking cessation process. Although there is limited evidence of their effectiveness, some people have found these methods helpful in reducing withdrawal symptoms and cravings. However, it is important to consider individual differences and to consult qualified health care professionals for individualized advice. In the following chapters, we will explore other strategies and tips to help you achieve your goal of a tobacco-free life.

CHAPTER 9: MANAGING WITHDRAWAL SYMPTOMS

When you quit smoking, you may experience a series of withdrawal symptoms that can make the process difficult. In this chapter, we'll look at these symptoms and provide practical tips for managing them effectively, to maximize your chances of success in quitting smoking.

9.1 Common withdrawal symptoms

Smoking cessation can cause a variety of physical and emotional symptoms. Here are some of the most common symptoms you may experience:

- Cravings: Cravings are one of the most common symptoms of withdrawal. They can occur at any time and vary in intensity. It is important to understand that cravings are temporary and will eventually diminish over time.

- Irritability and restlessness: Quitting smoking can upset your emotional balance, which can lead to irritability, restlessness and even anxiety. It is important to find stress management techniques to deal with these emotions.

- Physical Symptoms: You may experience physical symptoms such as headaches, fatigue, trouble sleeping, increased appetite, dizziness, increased coughing or a sore throat. These symptoms are temporary and are part of your body's healing process.

- Decreased concentration: Some smokers report a temporary decrease in their ability to concentrate and remember information. This may be because your brain is adjusting to the absence of nicotine.

9.2 Strategies for managing withdrawal symptoms

Fortunately, there are effective strategies for managing withdrawal symptoms and making them more bearable. Here are some practical tips:

- Adopt a healthy lifestyle: Maintaining a balanced diet, exercising regularly and getting enough sleep can help reduce withdrawal symptoms. These healthy habits also help build your physical and mental stamina.

- Find distractions: When you feel a craving, occupy your mind with distracting activities. This can be taking a walk, taking up a hobby, reading an interesting book or listening to soothing music.

- Use relaxation techniques: Relaxation can help calm irritability and agitation. Try deep breathing techniques, meditation, yoga or mindfulness practice to relax and calm down.

- Find social support: Talk to your friends and family about quitting smoking and seek social support. Join support groups, share your experiences and exchange tips with others who are going through the same thing. The support of others can play a crucial role in your success.

- Use nicotine replacement products: Nicotine replacement products, such as patches, gum or inhalers, can help reduce cravings and withdrawal symptoms. Talk to your health care provider to determine which option is right for you.

9.3 Be patient and persistent

It is important to remember that withdrawal symptoms are temporary and will gradually diminish as your body adjusts to the absence of nicotine. Be patient with yourself and don't get discouraged if you encounter difficulties. Continue to use the strategies that work for you and be proud of each step you take on your journey to a tobacco-free life.

In conclusion, managing withdrawal symptoms is an essential step in your quit smoking journey. By using stress management techniques, adopting a healthy lifestyle, finding distractions and seeking social support, you can minimize the impact of symptoms and increase your chances of success. In the following chapters, we will discuss other important aspects of your quitting journey.

CHAPTER 10: BUILDING MOTIVATION AND WILLPOWER

When you set out to quit smoking, it is essential to have strong motivation and willpower. In this chapter, we'll explore different strategies for strengthening your motivation and resolve to help you overcome challenges and maintain your commitment to a tobacco-free life.

10.1 Understanding your personal motivation

The first step in strengthening your motivation is to understand why you want to quit smoking. Take some time to think about your personal reasons. Is it to improve your health? Protect your loved ones from the dangers of second-hand smoke? Save money? Improve your appearance? Identify your deepest motivations and remind yourself of them regularly when you encounter difficulties.

10.2 Set clear and realistic goals

To maintain your motivation, it is important to set clear and realistic goals. Determine what you want to achieve and make a concrete plan of action. For example, set a quit date, define intermediate steps and reward yourself when you reach those goals. Having clear goals gives you direction and allows you to measure your progress.

10.3 Visualize your success

Visualization is a powerful technique for strengthening your motivation. Take a few moments each day to imagine your life as a non-smoker. Visualize yourself doing activities you enjoy, being healthy and feeling pride in your success in quitting smoking. This positive visualization strengthens your motivation and helps you stay focused on your goal.

10.4 Use positive affirmations

Positive affirmations are positive statements that you repeat to yourself regularly to boost your confidence and motivation. For example, tell yourself phrases such as "I am able to quit smoking," "I am determined to take care of my health," or "I am becoming a non-smoker. Repeat these statements every day to reinforce your positive mindset.

10.5 Finding Social Support

Social support is essential to strengthen your motivation and willpower. Talk to your friends and family about your quit process. Join support groups or group quitting programs. The support of others who are going through the same experience can encourage you, motivate you and give you a sense of belonging.

10.6 Avoiding risky situations

Identify risky situations that could compromise your motivation and willpower. For example, if you have a habit of smoking while drinking your morning coffee, consider changing your routine by having a cup of tea instead. Avoid places where you were tempted to smoke and stay away from smokers for a while. Create a supportive environment for your success.

10.7 Rewarding yourself

Reward yourself regularly when you reach milestones in your quitting journey. Set small rewards for yourself, such as buying something you like, planning a special outing, or giving yourself a moment of relaxation. These rewards boost your motivation and give you something to look forward to.

In conclusion, strengthening your motivation and willpower is crucial to your success in quitting smoking. By understanding your personal motivations, setting clear goals, using visualization and positive affirmation techniques, finding social support and avoiding risky situations, you can strengthen your resolve and increase your chances of success. Continue to remind yourself of the benefits of a tobacco-free life and be proud of every step you take toward this new reality.

CHAPTER 11:
AVOIDING PITFALLS
AND RELAPSE

When you quit smoking, it's important to stay alert and watch out for pitfalls and situations that could cause you to relapse. In this chapter, we'll look at the most common pitfalls you may face and provide practical tips for avoiding them, so you can maintain your commitment to a tobacco-free life.

11.1 Identify common pitfalls

It is essential to know the pitfalls that could lead you to relapse. Here are some of the most common pitfalls that quitters may face:

- Social situations: Social events, going out with friends, or parties can be challenging situations where the temptation to smoke may be present. It is important to be aware of these situations and to plan strategies to manage them.

- Stress: Stress can be a major trigger for cravings. When faced with stressful situations, it is important to find healthy ways to cope with stress, such as relaxation, exercise or meditation.

- Mental associations: After smoking for a long time, you may associate certain activities or times of day with smoking. For example, smoking after a meal or with a cup of coffee. It is crucial to break these mental associations by adopting new habits and finding healthy substitutes.

- Feelings of deprivation: Sometimes when you quit smoking, you may feel a sense of deprivation, as if you are depriving yourself of something enjoyable. It is important to change your perception and focus on the many benefits and freedoms you gain by being a non-smoker.

11.2 Develop avoidance strategies

Once you've identified potential pitfalls, it's time to develop strategies to avoid them. Here are some practical tips:

- Avoid risky situations: If you know that a particular situation may trigger a craving, avoid it as much as possible, at least in the early stages of your quit. If this is not possible, prepare yourself in advance with stress management techniques and healthy distractions.

- Use diversionary techniques: When you are tempted to smoke, find a diversionary activity to occupy your mind. This can be doing some breathing exercises, taking a brisk walk, reading an interesting book or listening to music.

- Find social support: Social support is valuable in preventing relapse. Talk openly about your quit process with family and friends or join a support group. Sharing your difficulties and receiving encouragement can help you stay motivated and avoid relapse.

- Learn to manage cravings: Cravings can be intense, but they are temporary. Learn techniques for managing cravings, such as deep breathing, progressive muscle relaxation or visualization. The more you practice these techniques, the better you will be able to control your cravings.

11.3 Deal with relapse with compassion

Despite your best efforts, you may experience a relapse. It is important to be compassionate with yourself and not judge yourself harshly. A relapse does not mean that you have failed, but simply that you have hit a roadblock. Recognize what led to the relapse, learn from it and get back on track with determination.

In conclusion, avoiding pitfalls and relapses is a key element in maintaining your commitment to a tobacco-free life. By identifying common pitfalls, developing avoidance strategies and finding social support, you increase your chances of success. Remember, every day without tobacco is a victory and you are well on your way to achieving your goal of a healthier, tobacco-free life.

CHAPTER 12: SOCIAL AND FAMILY SUPPORT

When you decide to quit smoking, social and family support can play a crucial role in your success. In this chapter, we'll explore the importance of social support, how to get it, and how to involve them in your quitting process.

12.1 Understand the importance of social support

Social support is essential when it comes to quitting a habit as difficult as smoking. It can help you stay motivated, overcome obstacles and maintain your commitment to a smoke-free life. Social support can come from your family, friends, co-workers or quit smoking support groups.

12.2 Communicate openly with those around you

The first step to getting social support is to communicate openly with those around you. Talk about your decision to quit smoking with your family, friends and loved ones. Tell them why it's important to you and how they can support you. Be honest about your challenges and concerns, and ask for their help and understanding.

12.3 Involve your family and friends

Your family and friends can play an active role in your quitting process. Here are some ways to get them involved:

- Ask them to be your allies: Ask your loved ones to be your allies in quitting smoking. They can encourage you, remind you why you decided to quit and help you avoid risky situations.

- Establish healthy routines together: Involve your family and friends in creating new healthy routines. For example, organize outings that don't involve smoking, play sports together or plan activities that are not associated with smoking.

- Find a Quit Partner: If someone close to you also smokes and wants to quit, consider supporting each other as quit partners. You can share your experiences, encourage each other and celebrate your successes together.

12.4 Joining support groups

Support groups are great resources for getting the social support you need as you quit smoking. Look for local support groups or online communities dedicated to quitting smoking. These groups provide a space where you can share your experiences, get practical advice and find the encouragement you need.

12.5 Using online applications and platforms

Apps and online platforms can also be great tools for social support. There are mobile apps specifically designed to help people quit smoking. They offer features such as progress tracking, tips, reminders and the ability to connect with others who are also trying to quit smoking.

In conclusion, social and family support is a key element in your quitting process. By communicating openly with those around you, by actively involving them in your process, by joining support groups and by using online applications and platforms, you surround yourself with a community of support that encourages and motivates you. Remember that you are not alone in your journey to quit smoking and that you have people ready to support you every step of the way.

CHAPTER 13:
ADOPTING NEW
LIFESTYLE HABITS

When you quit smoking, it's essential to adopt new lifestyle habits that promote a healthy life away from tobacco. In this chapter, we'll explore different habits you can incorporate into your daily life to strengthen your quitting process and help you maintain your commitment over the long term.

13.1 The importance of healthy living

Healthy lifestyle habits are an essential part of your quitting process. They help strengthen your overall health, reduce cravings and maintain your motivation. Adopting new positive habits will allow you to replace the old smoking habit with behaviors that are beneficial to your physical and mental well-being.

13.2 Make exercise part of your daily routine

Regular exercise can be a great help in quitting smoking. Not only does it help you reduce cravings, but it also improves your mood, energy and overall health. Try to fit at least 30 minutes of moderate to vigorous physical activity into your day. You can choose to walk, run, swim, bike or do anything else you enjoy. Find what works best for you and make it a regular habit.

13.3 Adopt a balanced diet

A balanced diet plays a key role in your quit smoking journey. Eat healthy, balanced meals that include fruits, vegetables, lean proteins and whole grains. Avoid processed foods that are high in sugar and fat. When you have a craving, choose healthy snacks such as fresh fruit, cut-up vegetables or nuts.

13.4 Manage stress in a healthy way

Stress can be a major trigger for cravings. Learn to manage stress in a healthy way by using relaxation techniques, such as meditation, deep breathing or yoga. Also find activities that help you relax and enjoy yourself, such as reading, listening to music, drawing or gardening. By incorporating relaxation and fun into your daily routine, you'll reduce stress and build resilience to cravings.

13.5 Getting enough sleep

Sleep is essential to your overall well-being and to maintaining your commitment to quitting smoking. Try to maintain a regular sleep routine and get enough sleep each night. Avoid screens before bedtime, create a sleep-friendly environment and practice relaxation techniques to help you fall asleep more easily. Quality sleep will help you be more energetic, focused and resistant to cravings.

13.6 Find new activities and hobbies

Replace the smoking habit with new activities and hobbies that give you pleasure. Find hobbies that stimulate your creativity, such as painting, dancing, photography or writing. Get involved in social activities, joining clubs or groups that share your interests. By exploring new passions and engaging in activities that you are passionate about, you will have less time and interest in smoking.

In conclusion, adopting new healthy lifestyle habits is essential to strengthen your quit smoking journey. By incorporating exercise, a balanced diet, stress management, adequate sleep and new activities into your daily routine, you will create an environment that is conducive to a tobacco-free life. These new habits will help you stay motivated, reduce cravings and maintain your commitment for the long term.

CHAPTER 14: MANAGING STRESS AND EMOTIONS WITHOUT TOBACCO

When quitting smoking, it is important to develop strategies for managing stress and emotions without resorting to smoking. In this chapter, we will explore different techniques and approaches to effectively manage stress and emotions, allowing you to maintain your quit smoking journey.

14.1 Understanding the link between tobacco, stress and emotions

It is common for smokers to use cigarettes as a way to cope with stress and negative emotions. However, it is important to understand that smoking does not actually solve these problems, but rather creates an addiction that makes the situation worse in the long run. By quitting smoking, you are giving yourself the opportunity to learn new and healthier ways of dealing with stress and emotions.

14.2 Practice stress management techniques

Stress management is essential to avoid the urge to smoke. There are many effective techniques for managing stress, including meditation, deep breathing, yoga, progressive muscle relaxation and visualization. Try different methods and find the one that works best for you. Practice these techniques regularly to reduce stress and increase your ability to cope with the challenges of life without tobacco.

14.3 Express your emotions in a healthy way

Quitting smoking can sometimes lead to an increase in emotions as you learn to cope with daily challenges without relying on cigarettes. Learn to express your emotions in healthy and constructive ways. You can write in a journal, talk to a trusted friend, engage in art activities, or attend support groups where you can share your experiences with others in a similar situation.

14.4 Adopt relaxation techniques

Relaxation techniques are a great way to deal with stress and emotions without tobacco. Try relaxing activities such as taking a hot bath, listening to soothing music, walking in nature, gardening or reading a good book. Take time to relax each day and make it a priority in your schedule.

14.5 Exercise regularly

Regular exercise is not only good for your physical health, but also for your mental and emotional well-being. When you exercise, your body releases endorphins, chemicals that improve your mood and reduce stress. Choose a physical activity that you enjoy, such as walking, running, dancing, swimming or cycling, and do it regularly. You'll find that regular exercise helps you manage emotions and maintain your commitment to a tobacco-free life.

14.6 Finding Social Support

Social support is essential for coping with stress and emotions during your quitting process. Surround yourself with positive, encouraging people who support you in your decision to quit. Join support groups, attend group therapy sessions, or use online apps and platforms that offer support and advice. Talking about your feelings with others who understand what you are going through can be very beneficial.

In conclusion, managing stress and emotions without tobacco is essential to maintaining your quit process. By using stress management techniques, expressing your emotions in healthy ways, adopting relaxation techniques, exercising regularly and finding social support, you will strengthen your ability to cope with life's challenges without resorting to smoking. Continue to explore different approaches and find the ones that work best for you.

CHAPTER 15: MAINTAINING FREEDOM: PREVENTING RELAPSE

Once you have successfully quit smoking, it is important to take steps to maintain your freedom from tobacco and prevent relapse. In this final chapter, we'll explore strategies and tips for strengthening your quitting process and avoiding a relapse to smoking.

15.1 Understanding the risk factors for relapse

It is essential to understand the risk factors for relapse in order to better anticipate them and take preventive measures. Some common factors include stress, social situations, sudden cravings, memories associated with smoking and negative emotions. Identify the risk factors that affect you personally and be prepared to deal with them proactively.

15.2 Strengthen your coping skills

One of the keys to preventing relapse is developing strong coping skills. Learn stress management, problem-solving and decision-making strategies to deal with challenges that arise. The more you feel you can cope with difficult situations without resorting to smoking, the more resistant you will be to temptations and cravings.

15.3 Avoiding Triggers

Identify the triggers that cause you to smoke and take steps to avoid them whenever possible. This may include social situations where others are smoking, places where you have a habit of smoking, smoking-related activities, or particular times of stress. If you can't avoid certain triggers completely, plan alternative strategies for dealing with them, such as practicing relaxation techniques or using nicotine replacement products.

15.4 Maintain a healthy lifestyle

A healthy lifestyle is essential to maintaining your freedom from tobacco. Continue to eat a balanced diet, exercise regularly and manage stress in a healthy way. Also, make sure you get enough sleep and take care of your mental health by engaging in activities that give you pleasure and well-being. A healthy body and mind build resilience to cravings.

15.5 Coping with potential relapses

Despite your best efforts, you may experience a relapse. If this happens, don't be discouraged and don't consider it a failure. Instead, use this experience as an opportunity to learn and strengthen your resolve to quit smoking. Analyze the circumstances that led to the relapse and think of strategies to avoid them in the future. Don't hesitate to ask for support from those around you, join a support group or consult a health care professional.

15.6 Celebrate your successes

Remember to celebrate each step in your journey to becoming smoke-free. Whether it's a week, a month, a year or more, every day without tobacco is a victory. Reward yourself in a way that is not related to smoking, such as going out with friends, relaxing, or buying a treat for yourself. Celebrating your successes motivates you and reminds you why you chose to go tobacco-free.

In conclusion, maintaining your freedom from tobacco and preventing relapse takes vigilance and commitment. By understanding risk factors, building coping skills, avoiding triggers, maintaining a healthy lifestyle, dealing with potential relapses and celebrating your successes, you will be able to stay on the path to a tobacco-free life. Remember, you are capable of living a full and healthy life free of tobacco.

CONCLUSION

Congratulations on reading "Freedom Regained: The Best Methods for Quitting Smoking"! You've taken the first step toward a smoke-free life and the freedom to choose your health and well-being.

In this book, we've explored the different aspects of quitting smoking, from the dangers of smoking to effective ways to quit. You've learned about the harmful effects of smoking on your health, as well as the underlying reasons why you made the decision to say goodbye to this harmful habit.

We discussed the importance of setting realistic goals, preparing yourself mentally, choosing the method that works best for you and managing withdrawal symptoms. We also covered topics such as strengthening motivation, relapse prevention, social support and adopting new healthy lifestyle habits.

Remember that every journey to quit smoking is unique, and it is normal to encounter challenges along the way. However, you now have the knowledge, tools and strategies to overcome these obstacles and maintain your commitment to a tobacco-free life.

The key to success is your determination, will and perseverance. Be compassionate with yourself, be patient and don't be afraid to ask for support when you need it. You are not alone in this journey, many people have successfully quit smoking and lived a healthier and more fulfilling life.

Also remember the benefits that await you as a former smoker. Your health will improve, your breath will be easier, your sense of smell and taste will awaken, and you will feel proud of your accomplishment. Every day without tobacco is a victory, so celebrate every step of your journey.

As I conclude this book, I encourage you to continue to cultivate your freedom from tobacco. Stay motivated, adopt strategies to deal with challenges, and make your health and well-being a priority. You have made the choice to take back control of your life, and that opens the door to a brighter, healthier future.

Goodbye to tobacco and hello to newfound freedom!